Mazen Almasri

Bone graft for future dental implants, the truthful reality

Mazen Almasri

Bone graft for future dental implants, the truthful reality

Is Bone ceramic® an osteoconductive material when used as an onlay graft?

LAP LAMBERT Academic Publishing

Impressum / Imprint

Bibliografische Information der Deutschen Nationalbibliothek: Die Deutsche Nationalbibliothek verzeichnet diese Publikation in der Deutschen Nationalbibliografie; detaillierte bibliografische Daten sind im Internet über http://dnb.d-nb.de abrufbar.
Alle in diesem Buch genannten Marken und Produktnamen unterliegen warenzeichen-, marken- oder patentrechtlichem Schutz bzw. sind Warenzeichen oder eingetragene Warenzeichen der jeweiligen Inhaber. Die Wiedergabe von Marken, Produktnamen, Gebrauchsnamen, Handelsnamen, Warenbezeichnungen u.s.w. in diesem Werk berechtigt auch ohne besondere Kennzeichnung nicht zu der Annahme, dass solche Namen im Sinne der Warenzeichen- und Markenschutzgesetzgebung als frei zu betrachten wären und daher von jedermann benutzt werden dürften.

Bibliographic information published by the Deutsche Nationalbibliothek: The Deutsche Nationalbibliothek lists this publication in the Deutsche Nationalbibliografie; detailed bibliographic data are available in the Internet at http://dnb.d-nb.de.
Any brand names and product names mentioned in this book are subject to trademark, brand or patent protection and are trademarks or registered trademarks of their respective holders. The use of brand names, product names, common names, trade names, product descriptions etc. even without a particular marking in this works is in no way to be construed to mean that such names may be regarded as unrestricted in respect of trademark and brand protection legislation and could thus be used by anyone.

Coverbild / Cover image: www.ingimage.com

Verlag / Publisher:
LAP LAMBERT Academic Publishing
ist ein Imprint der / is a trademark of
AV Akademikerverlag GmbH & Co. KG
Heinrich-Böcking-Str. 6-8, 66121 Saarbrücken, Deutschland / Germany
Email: info@lap-publishing.com

Herstellung: siehe letzte Seite /
Printed at: see last page
ISBN: 978-3-659-39682-3

Zugl. / Approved by: Montreal, McGill University, Diss., 2009

Copyright © 2013 AV Akademikerverlag GmbH & Co. KG
Alle Rechte vorbehalten. / All rights reserved. Saarbrücken 2013

TABLE OF CONTENT

Acknowledgement ...3

CHAPTER ONE (INTRODUCTION AND BACKGROUND: PRINCIPLES OF BONE GRAFTING) ...4

Introduction
Bone augmentation principles
Inlay vs onlay graft
Guided bone regeneration
Non resorbable membranes
Resorbable membranes
Summary

CHAPTER TWO (PROSPECTIVE EXPIREMENTAL STUDY: MATERIALS AND METHODS) ...16

Experimental Model
Treatment group
Experiment Armamentarium
Preparation and Anesthetic Technique
Operative Procedure
Post Operative Care
Post-Mortem Assessment
Samples extract
Micro-CT analysis
Histology
Histomorphometry

CHAPTER THREE (STUDY RESULTS) ...27
Clinical Course
Gross description
Micro CT
Histology
Histomorphometry

CHAPTER FOUR (DISCUSSION AND CONCLUSION) ...37
Biodegradable membrane
Test group (Bone Ceramic)
Control group (Empty chambers)
Conclusion and recommendation

OTHERS:
Appendices 40
References 46

ACKNOWLEDGEMENTS

Between the training programs, hospitals, and faculty teaching, we always forget that sharing the knowledge is one of the greatest honors that any scientist can do. It is true, I might be doing that probably every day in my life, but I still have to thank some of my great friends and students whom influenced me toward sharing this project in the this format, a book. I hope that the readers can find in this book what they need about the major principles of bone grafting techniques and what is needed to help them perform further prospective projects in this field.

In addition, I would like to express my gratitude to the following:

1- **Dr. Timothy Head**; my mentor in the field of Oral Maxillofacial Surgery in McGill University for his continuous support and supervision throughout the training program in McGill University Health Center and the research projects in the department.

2- My colleagues **Dr. Abdullah Alharkan** and **Dr. Badr Aljandan** for their advices and ideas.

3- *F.O.R.C.E Alumni Foundation* for their financial assistance toward research

4- **Stryker** Company for providing the needed armamentarium.

5- McGill University **Bone Biology Lab** and Montreal General Hospital **Research Center/ operating theatre** for their cooperation throughout the project.

6- **Dr. Mustafa Altalibi**, DMD, McGill Faculty of Dentistry; for his help in samples collection and analysis.

7- Last but not least, to the **Ministry of Higher Education** in Saudi Arabia for their continuous support toward advancing the health care and medical education.

CHAPTER ONE
INTRODUCTION AND BACKGROUND; PRINCIPLES OF BONE GRAFTING

INTRODUCTION AND BACKGROUND:

Dental implant placement is frequently challenged by deficiency of bone volume in the horizontal and/or vertical dimensions. This deficiency is due to atrophy, periodontal disease, trauma, pathology, or infections *(Barber and Betts 1993)*. Reconstruction of the alveolar ridge has been attempted using various methods such as autogenous bone grafts, allogenic bone grafts, xenografts, alloplasts, and the concept of guided bone regeneration (GBR) *(Norton et al. 2003)*. Autogenous bone has generally been considered to be the gold standard for alveolar ridge reconstruction due to its unique osteogenic, osteoconductive, osteoinductive, and continuous remodeling capabilities *(Moy and Aghaloo 2007)*. However, autogenous bone grafts have some disadvantages such as, donor site morbidity, limited quantity, and rapid resorption rate when compared to non autogenous grafts *(Albrektsson and Johansson 2001)*. These drawbacks were the reasons to investigate other options such as hydroxyapatite (HA) and calcium phosphate compounds *(Constantz 1998)*. HA and calcium phosphates represents the core of Bone Ceramic alloplastic grafts, which is one material that will be discussed in detail in this article *(Almasri and Altalibi 2011)*.

Bone augmentation principles:
It is important to define some of the fundamentals of bone grafting and alveolar reconstruction. These fundamentals will help the operator to customize a proper treatment for each case.

" Bone Graft Incorporation " is defined as the fusion of the bone graft to the recipient site, which is followed by bone remodeling and eventually formation of more mature bone, thereafter enabling the bone graft to withstand continuous functional loading *(El-Hakim 2006)*.

Osteogenesis is defined as the formation of new bone from osteoprogenitor cells. The osteoprogenitor cells either arise from the recipient site or are transplanted into the wound by the graft material. Autogenous bone graft is an example of osteogenic materials.

Osteoinduction refers to the ability of the graft to stimulate mesenchymal stem cell differentiation to osteoblasts. These mesenchymal cells are triggered by other osteoprogenitor cells and growth factors like bone morphogenic proteins (BMP), platelet derived growth factor (PDGF), and TGF-B.

Osteoconduction is the process by which a bone graft material provides a scaffold into which blood vessels and cells can migrate. Bone Ceramic is an example of osteoconductive materials *(Aljandan 2007)*.

Autogenous Bone graft: Evidence confirms that autogenous bone is the gold standard bone augmentation material due to its unique osteogenic, osteoinductive, osteoconductive and continuous remodeling capabilities *(Moy and Aghaloo 2007, Aljandan 2007)*. Studies have shown that the implant success in autogenous bone grafts is generally over 95%; however, success has varied from 70 to 100% depending on the inclusion criteria of each study *(Barber and Betts 1993, Hallman et al 2002)*. Factors affecting implant success are the quality of bone, patient health status, degree of bone loss before implant placement, smoking, clenching, bruxism, and the operator expertise *(Hallman et al 2002)*.

Autogenous bone grafts can be harvested from intraoral or extraoral sites. The amount of autogenous bone required can be a determining factor of the graft harvest site. Intraoral sites are usually used to reconstruct smaller areas, i.e. for placing one or two implants. Autografts can be harvested intraorally from the maxillary tuberosity, chin, external oblique ridge, and coronoid process. Moreover, extraoral donor sites can provide larger quantities of autogenous bone compared to intraoral harvest sites. The most common extraoral harvest sites are: tibial plateau (provides 25-40cc of uncompressed cancellous bone), anterior iliac crest (50-75cc), and posterior iliac crest (100-120cc) *(Yildirim et al. 2000)*. The main disadvantages of using autogenous bone grafts are: second operative site morbidity and increased operation time *(Norton et al. 2003, Leonetti & Koup 2003)*. Another significant consideration in autografts is their rapid resorbability, which accounts for 30 to 55% during the first six months of healing and proceeds in a slower rate thereafter *(Johansson et al 2001)*. The idea of using calvarial bone grafts has been proposed and proven to have less resorption rate, during the first 6 months of healing, due to its intramembraneous ossification origin *(Jensen & Sindet 1991)*.

Allografts are tissues derived from one human, and following processing are grafted into another human. The stated advantages of allografts are their osteoconductive properties and the possibility that they are osteoinductive secondary to the presence of bone morphogenic protein (BMP) traces. These BMP traces act as the major cytokine regulating bone induction *(Moghadam et al. 2004)*. Despite this, their osteoinductive property is inferior to fresh autogenous bone grafts. A major disadvantage in using allografts is the risk of infectious disease transmission; however, this risk is minimized following the advancements in drug and pharmaceutical materials processing *(Yildirim et al. 2000)*. It is therefore necessary to discuss these facts with the patients in order to clarify any religious or personal objections.

Xenografts are grafts derived from different species other than human (e.g Bovine), and processed to be used in humans. A xenograft acts as an osteoconductive material and has the advantage of unlimited quantity *(Tuominen et al. 2001)*. The main disadvantage of using xenografts is the prolonged resorption period, which requires a waiting period of 9 to 12 months before attempting an implant placement *(Alharkan 2007)*.

Alloplastic grafts are inorganic synthetic materials that have the advantage of being osteoconductive, synthetic origin, and availability in unlimited quantity. Variable mixtures have been studied in the literature, and calcium phosphate represents one of the most commonly studied ones *(Jensen et al. 2001)*.

Calcium phosphate alloplast is a generic term that consists of the chemical formulations; $CaOH - 3(PO_4) - H_2O$. This chemical formula can experience a transformation from a liquid or pasty state to a solid state, in which the end-product of the reaction is calcium phosphate. Calcium phosphate grafts consist generally of a concentrated mixture of one or several calcium phosphate powders and an aqueous solution (e.g. water) *(Constantz BR et al. 1998)*. These alloplasts have excellent tissue compatibility and osteoconductive capabilities *(Damien and Parsons 1991)*. Furthermore, hydroxyapatite (HA; $Ca_5 - (PO_4)_3 - OH$) is a crystalline example that has been studied since 1970, and clinically applied as a biomaterial substitute to repair craniofacial defects *(Shindo M et al. 1993)*. Moreover, Gosain et al *(2002)* claimed HA to possess osteoinductive potential when HA grafts were placed into soft tissue pockets in sheep and further bone formation was achieved in these pockets. The exact mechanism of this osteoinductive potential has not been understood. HA's osteoconductivity has been proven by the successful filling of calvarial bone defects in sheep. Gossain et al reported that the ceramic form of HA has more potential for bone replacement than the cement form, and that the major disadvantages of HA are their brittleness and low degradation potential *(Gossain et al 2002, Bohner M 2007)*.

The material of interest in our experiment is alloplastic in nature such as Bone Ceramic® (BC). BC is an alloplastic material composed of a combination of HA (Ca_5-$(PO_4)_3$-OH); 60% and beta tricalcium phosphate (bTCP; Ca_3-$(PO_4)_2$); 40%. Unlike other calcium phosphates, Straumann® BC is not simply a mixture of HA and bTCP, it is chemically synthesized as a composite to ensure homogenous distribution of the two components. Its composition of HA and bTCP gives it two phases of activity: first, it supports the bulk of the graft by the hard HA particles; and second, it enhances the subsequent replacement of the bTCP degradation products with blood vessels and mature lamellar bone by the faster resorption rate of bTCP compared to HA *(Gosain 2004, Nakadate M et al 2008)*. Jensen SS et al *(2006)* studied the resorption pattern of bTCP by creating bony defects on minipig mandibular angles and grafting these defects with bTCP. Subsequently, the subjects were sacrificed at 1, 2, 4, and 8 weeks respectively in order to analyze the grafts' histologic and histomorphometric characteristics. Significant resorption was noticed throughout the periods, and mulltinucleated giant cells were noticed actively engulfing the dissolved bTCP particles. This analysis indicated that degradation of bTCP seems to be a combination of dissolution and direct cell-mediated resorption.

BC is 90% porous, with pores sizes ranging between 100 to 500 microns in diameter. This high porosity allows maximum space for vascularization, macrophage invasion, osteoblast migration and bone deposition, of which the exact mechanism is not completely understood. Studies have shown that bone morphogenic protein (transforming growth factor – beta (TGF-β) superfamily), derived from platelets and the surrounding tissues, is a possible molecular initiator that may regulate cartilage and bone differentiation in vivo *(Pollick et al. 1995)*. The provider suggests more than 6 months of waiting period before placing an implant in Bone Ceramic grafts.

Inlay versus onlay bone graft healing:

Inlay bone grafting is defined as the procedure where the graft material is placed into a native contained bony cavity *(Elhakim 2006)*, while onlay bone grafting is the procedure where the graft material is placed on top of a flat bony surface. It is well known that inlay bone grafts are more predictable than onlays, due to the presence of multiple walls that contain the graft and provide osteoprogenitor cells and nutrients *(Ozaki and Buchman 1998)*. Therefore, inlay grafts exhibit increased volume with time, in contrast to onlay grafts which resorb over time *(Rosenthal and Buchman 2003) (Marx et al. 1993, 2002)*.

The use of BC as an inlay graft has been previously discussed in the literature. *Ellinger et al (1986)* showed promising results when BC was used to reconstruct periodontal defects, and *Fleckenstein KB et al (2006)* showed significant new bone formation when BC was used to reconstruct iatrogenically created calvarial bone defects in rats. *Froum S et al* used histomorphometry to compare BC and anorganic bovine bone (ABM) for sinus lift grafting. Six to eight months post grafting; a core of the graft was harvested from twenty one healed sinuses and sent for histomorphometric analysis. The results comparing BC and ABM showed an average vital bone content of 28.35% and 22.27%, respectively. The average percentage of residual graft particles was 28.4% in the BC cores and 26.0% in the ABM cores. The difference in vital bone formation was not statistically significant between sinuses treated with the BC and sinuses treated with the ABM; therefore, both materials appeared to be osteoconductive.

The use of BC as an onlay graft was studied by *Gosain et al (2005)*. Gosain et al compared facial augmentations in ten sheep using autogenous calvarial bone and HA derived biomaterials including BC. 16.8 x 5mm blocks were fabricated and implanted on different locations on sheep faces and craniums. One year later, samples were harvested for volume analysis and the results showed that BC blocks exhibited more predictable graft volumes than autogenous calvarial blocks, which demonstrated significant volume reduction ($P < 0.0001$).

Guided bone regeneration:

Guided bone regeneration (GBR) is defined as the process of applying a functional matrix or creating a space under occlusive barriers in order to selectively allow for bone forming cells to produce bone uniquely. The periosteum has an important role in bone regeneration as it is composed of an outer fibrous (vascular) layer and an inner cambium (osteogenic) layer. Kostopoulos and Karring *(1995)* evaluated the bone-forming capacity of the outer (fibrous) and inner (cambium) layer of the mandibular periosteum in skeletally mature rats. Their experiment was carried out in 25 rats, where the mandibular ramus was exposed on one side (experimental side) after elevating a muscle-periosteal flap. Next, a teflon capsule was placed with its opening facing the periosteum, at the subsurface of the raised muscle-periosteal flap, and sutures were used to fix the capsule in place. In the contralateral side, the periosteum of the lateral aspect was left intact on the ramus and a teflon capsule was placed with its opening facing the periosteum. The histological analysis demonstrated that all the experiment and control specimens revealed some bone production 7 days after the operation. At 120 days, the mean amount of new bone produced in the experimental capsules was merely 3% (range 0-15%) of the total space created by the capsule, while it was 68% (range 41-85%) for the control capsules. The results demonstrated that substantial amounts of bone can be produced by the placement of an occlusive teflon capsule facing a mandible covered with periosteum *(Kostopoulos and Karring 1995)*.

It has been proven that the periosteum has an important role as an occlusive barrier. *Adeyemo W et al (2008)* examined the role of the host periosteum on the healing of an onlay graft to the mandible based on histologic and immunohistochemical analysis. Twelve adult sheep were used in the study and all received four iliac corticocancellous onlay bone grafts on the lateral surface of the mandible. In group 1, the block graft was placed in direct contact with the recipient cortical bed and fixed with micro-screws, and in group 2, the recipient cortical bed was perforated before graft placement. The host periosteum around the graft was excised before flap replacement in group 3, and in group 4, a sheet of silicone membrane was placed between the graft and the recipient bed. The animals were sacrificed at 4, 8, 12 and 16 weeks postoperatively. Samples were harvested and sent for histology and immunohistochemistry for proliferation and apoptotic markers. The results indicated that recipient cortical bed perforations offered no advantage over the non-perforated bed regarding healing and integration of the bone graft. Excision of the host's overlying periosteum was accompanied with rapid resorption of the grafts and partial or complete replacement with fibrous connective tissue (group 3). Infiltration of the graft by connective tissue in group 3 demonstrated that the absence of periosteum lead to infiltration of the graft site by non-osteogenic cells. Total or partial replacement of the graft with connective tissue was observed only in group 3.

Types of GBR materials:

Different types of GBR membranes are available in clinical practice. The criteria to assess GBR membranes are biocompatibility, resorbability, support of the underlying graft, exclusion of the undesired non-osteoprogenitor cells, and ease of manipulation. However, it is difficult to find a single material that contains all the ideal criteria *(McAllister et al. 2007)*. Two major categories of membranes are available in practice, resorbable and non resorbable.

A- Non Resorbable membranes: Examples of non resorbable membranes are polytetrafluoroethylene (ePTFE), titanium reinforced ePTFE, and titanium mesh. The ePTFE was one of the original materials used for this purpose. The major disadvantage of ePTFE is that once it is exposed by wound dehiscence, the infection rate is high. In addition, ePTFE will not support epithelialization and granulation on top of the exposed surface, consequently this will usually require preterm removal *(Buser et. al. 1993, 1995; Bartee 1995)*.

Titanium mesh is another example of non resorbable products which has the following advantages;
- Biocompatibility
- Easy of manipulation
- Excellent support to the underlying graft
- Low graft-resorption rate *(Von Arx et al. 1996, 1998)*.

The chief disadvantage of titanium meshes is that they do not resorb. Hence, 3 to 5 months after placement, titanium meshes should be removed in order to place dental implants. The process of removal of these titanium meshes is usually traumatic to the bone graft and the soft tissue flap; therefore caution should be taken while doing so. Another disadvantage of using a titanium mesh is that healing by secondary intention is unlikely to occur if the titanium surface is exposed by wound dehiscence.

B- Resorbable Membranes: The term biodegradation is used to explain the course of resorption/ degradation of these membranes in the human body. Two major categories of resorbable membranes are available for clinical use, synthetic and natural products. Variable thicknesses are available, ranging from 0.05 mm to 1.5 mm, which lead to variable biodegradation time frames ranging from 3 to 36 weeks. The natural products are usually composed of animal type-one collagen, which can be extracted from animals' Achilles tendon. These natural products are biodegraded by enzymatic biochemical processes. The main disadvantage of a collagen membrane is the lack of strength to support a particulate graft.

The other category of resorbable membranes is the synthetically fabricated ones. There are variable copolymers made of polylactic acid (PLA) and polyglycolic acid (PGA) monomers. It is imperative to understand that each copolymer has different characteristics and biological responses depending on its manufacturing process (crystallization degree, reticulation level, etc.) and not only on its chemical composition. For example, PLA polymers produce inflammatory effects and have long degradation times that can reach over 5 years; conversely the copolymer PLA/PGA has appreciable osteoconductivity, absence of an inflammatory response, and better solubility than PLA or PGA individually *(Kontino et al. 2005)*. The copolymer PLA/PGA has good solubility in most of the common solvents including chlorinated solvents, tetrahydrofuran, acetone or ethyl acetate. PLA/PGA is degraded via hydrolysis in the body to produce the original monomers, lactic acid (LA) and glycolic acid (GA). The final by products of PLA/PGA degradation are water and carbon dioxide *(Meadows 1993, McAllister et al. 2007)*. The main advantage of a PLA/PGA membrane over a collagen membrane is better stability.

Variable PLA/PGA products have been investigated such as bone plates *(Ferretti et al. 2002, Landes 2003, Eppley 2004)*, socket preservation sponges *(Sireno et al. 2003) (Rimondini et al. 2005)*, bony defect fillers *(Imbronito et al 2005)*, and resorbable screws. Resorbable screws have been used successfully for bone graft block fixation. Their main advantage in this application is avoiding subsequent screw removal, compared to titanium screws *(Chacon GE et al 2004)*.

Resorbable PLA/PGA membranes are used for guided bone regeneration and as bone graft carriers; therefore *Kinoshita Y et al (1993)* studied the geometry maintenance capability of PLA membranes. The experiment was done on a canine model where cylindrical PLA carriers were fabricated and filled up with autogenous bone and then placed subcutaneousely. In 3 months, 80% of the carrier geometry was maintained. These same authors published another study in 1997, in which they studied bone volume maintenance in PLA carriers placed into iatrogenically created mandibular continuity defects. Iliac crest bone grafts were harvested and packed into U-shaped PLA carriers that were fixed to the superior border of the mandible in an inverted U-shape fashion. Canines were scarified at 3, 6, and 12 months respectively for graft volume analysis. Results showed predictable bone volume maintenance in the trays; therefore the authors concluded that PLA carriers were efficient bone graft carrier devices.

Studies have shown that PLA/PGA membranes are biocompatible and can provide stable wound healing. *Eppley et al (1997)* demonstrated stable wound healing when a PLA/PGA mesh was used to stabilize calvarial bone grafts. It was reported that it took 9 months for the PLA/PGA membrane to completely degrade. *Nieminen et al (2006)* studied the PLA/PGA degradation rate in a prospective study, where Inion® membranes were fixed into the lateral aspect of the mandible of sheep. The animals were sacrificed at 6, 12, 26, 52 and 104 weeks postoperatively. At 6–26 weeks, the mesh was present and surrounded by a fibrous connective tissue network. At 52-104 weeks, neither the mesh, the fibrous networks, nor any foreign body reactions were detected. These authors concluded that complete degradation of the PLA/PGA membranes is to be expected 12 months post implantation.

Summary:

Dental implants have become one of the most important interventions in the field of Oral Maxillofacial reconstruction. Proper implant placement is mandatory to achieve optimal results; however, this is frequently challenged by alveolar bone deficiency. Alveolar bone reconstruction is often needed before dental implant treatment, which can be in the form of inlay or onlay bone grafting. It is well known that the onlay bone grafting procedure is more challenging than inlay grafting. Autogenous bone grafts are considered to be the best grafting materials; despite this, the surgeon may encounter variable situations when he/she has to use non autogenous bone substitutes; therefore we are investigating the option of using BC, an alloplastic material. Our aim is to know if BC is an osteoconductive material when used as an onlay graft under a PLA/PGA membrane.

CHAPTER TWO
PROSPECTIVE EXPIREMENT: MATERIALS AND METHODS

EXPERIMENTAL MODEL:

Adult female New Zealand White (NZW) rabbits, weighing 3.0 to 4.0 kg, obtained from the Charles River breeding facility, were used as the experimental animals. The NZW rabbit has been used extensively as a model for bone grafting experiments in the maxillofacial skeleton. The rabbits' bone remodeling cycle is short (sigma = 6 weeks) while for humans the sigma value is 17 weeks. Using the sigma ratio between human and rabbit, conclusions can be extrapolated from the rabbit model to human equivalents *(Roberts et al. 1998)*.

TREATMENT GROUPS

Eleven New Zealand white rabbits were used. On each rabbit's mandible, one test sample (BC chamber) was placed on the (right or left) body, while the control sample (empty, E chamber) was placed on the contralateral side. Randomization in placing the samples between the right and left bodies of the mandible were applied and identified. The Bone Ceramic graft was packed into the PLA/PGA chamber which was fixed to the mandible using 3 to 4 titanium screws (Figures 1, 2, 3). Before fixating the chamber, two bleeding points were made through the cortex of the mandible using a bone tap driver, in order to expose the chambers' inner space to bone marrow. The sample size for this experiment was calculated by Professor Jose Corea (McGill University Statistics Department), using the data of Aljandan's (2007) MSc thesis – McGill, Alharkan's (2007) MSc thesis – McGill, and the "Simple Sample Size Calculator" software. We chose a power of 80% to prove effectiveness, a standard deviation of 1.5 and a total confidence width of 2.5. The required sample size was found to be twelve rabbits (N= 12), thus, twelve rabbits were ordered. One was eliminated due to aberrant reaction to preoperative anesthetic medication; hence, the remaining animals were numbered subsequently from 1 to 11.

EXPERIMENT ARMAMENTARIUM

Biodegradable mesh:

Preparation of the membrane was done following the manufacturer's instruction. The manufacturer's plasticizer, N-Methyl-Pyrolidone (NMP) a widely used solvent for water insoluble drugs, was used to soften a 0.2 mm dense PLA/PGA membrane *(Inion GTR^{TM} Finland)*. Subsequently, the softened form was molded to the desired shape by press forming the material over a metallic template. The metallic chamber had a total volume of 48 mm^3 and a dimension of 4x4x3 mm. The molded Inion membrane had an approximate dimension of 4.5x4.5x3.2 mm and resulted in a chamber volume of 64.8 mm^3 (Figures 2, 3).

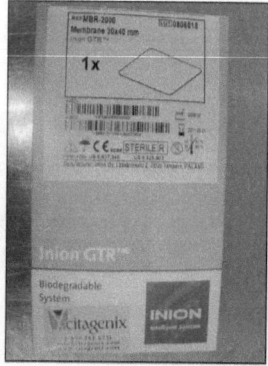
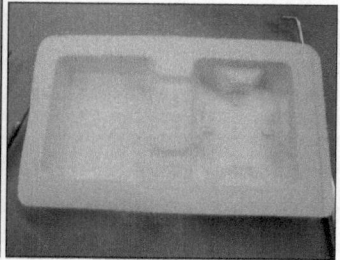

Figure-1: Inion™ biodegradable membrane is immersed completely in the plasticizer (right).

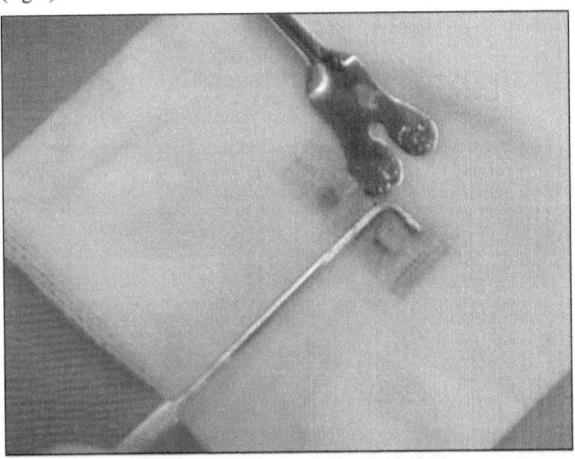

Figure - 2: After the plasticizing step, molding the membrane over the metallic template

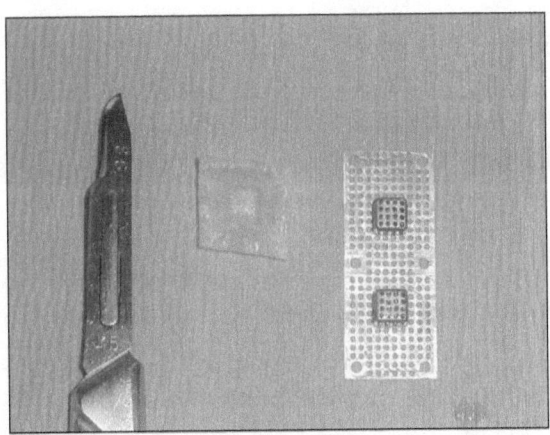

Figure - 3: The chamber in the middle showing the replica size to the metal chamber on the right. Notice the size relative to #15 blade.

PREPARATION AND ANESTHETIC TECHNIQUE

To reduce variability, all the operative procedures were performed by one surgeon and all animal handling such as injections and anesthesia were performed by the Montreal General Hospital (MGH) Animal Health Technical Team. All the manipulations and procedures performed on the rabbits were approved by the McGill University Veterinarian Committee and the McGill University Animal Ethics Committee (Appendix III).

To acclimatize the animals, all of them were kept in a designated room at the MGH research institute and a period of seven to ten days was allowed between the purchase time and the surgery date. The animals were housed in individual cages and were given water and food. One animal developed an aberrant reaction to a preoperative anesthetic drug and was eliminated from the study.

Water and food were withheld from each animal 12 hours prior to the surgery. At one hour pre-operatively, each animal was sedated by injecting Butorphanol 0.3 mg/kg intra-muscularly. Thereafter, the animal was brought to the operating room, where intravenous access was established by inserting a 22 gauge catheter into the auricular vein, and general anesthesia was induced using the combination of drugs: Thiopental (25 mg/kg), Xylazin (1-3 mg/kg), Atropin (1 mg/kg), and Ketamin (35-50 mg/kg). These drugs were injected intravenously and thereafter, the rabbit was intubated using a pediatric, uncuffed, endotracheal tube. General anesthesia was then maintained using a 2-4% of Isoflurane inhalation agent and the animal was connected to a mechanical ventilator (on an assisted ventilation mode) for the entire duration of the surgery. At the same time, all the monitoring devices, a pulse oximeter and a thermometer, were also connected. Each animal received a preoperative dose of antibiotic (Cefazolin 12.5 mg/kg) intravenousely (Novopharm Ltd., Toronto, Canada).

OPERATIVE PROCEDURE

The same technique was applied to all the animals, in which the first animal was labeled as number 1, and the last animal as number 11. Just prior to the surgery, the skin over submandibular area was shaved and disinfected using Povidine solution.

The animal was then placed on one lateral side and the surgical site was prepped and draped. A 3 cm submandibular skin incision was made along the inferior border of the mandible and carried through skin, subcutaneous tissue, muscle, and periosteum, to expose the inferior border of the mandiblular body. This was followed by a subperiosteal dissection along the lateral aspect of the mandible's body (Figures 4, 5, 6). Following the manufacturer's recommendations, Bone Ceramic material was wet with 0.9% normal saline, to ease its manipulation (Figure 7), and was packed gently into one chamber without excessive crushing force. The chamber was applied above the two cortical bleeding points and secured to one body of the mandible using 3 to 4 titanium screws (4-6 mm long/ 1.7 mm diameter). The periostium was protected and kept intact, then carefully laid over the chambers. The incision was closed in layers starting with the periostium and muscle over the chamber using 3-0 Vicryl suture in tension free - continuous fashion. Next, the skin was closed using 3-0 Monocryl suture in similar continuous fashion. Subsequently, the rabbit was turned onto the other side to perform placement of the control sample (empty chamber) using the same operative technique.

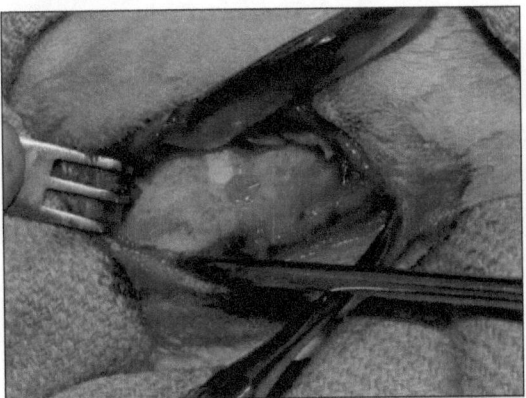

Figure - 4: Exposure of lateral aspect of the mandible's body

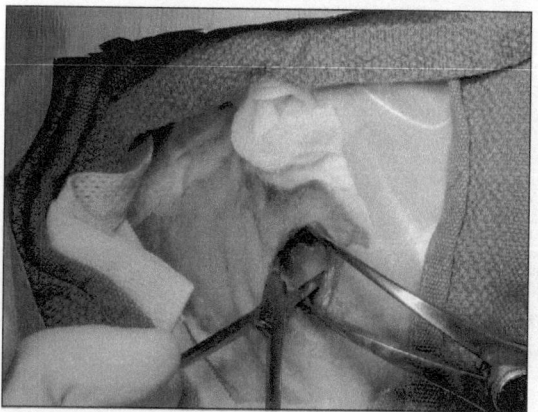

Figure – 5: Another mandible exposure and adapting the chamber onto the mandibular body.

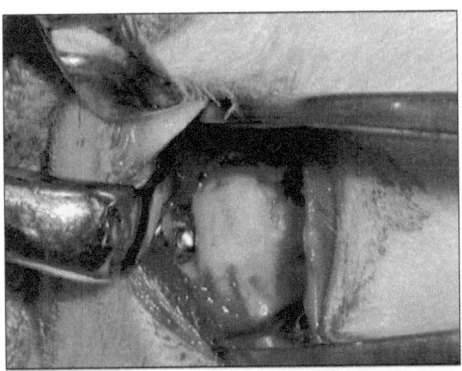

Figure – 6: The chamber fixed to body with screws.

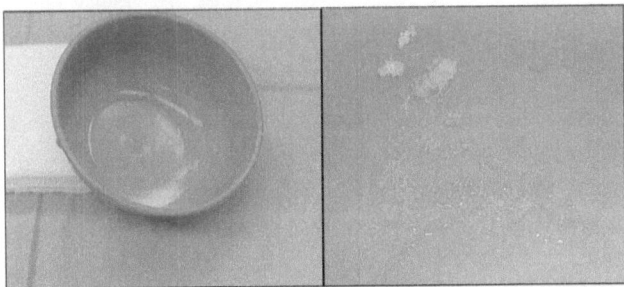

Figure- 7: The white BC white particles placed into a green dish (Left). A sample of BC wet with normal saline and became ready to be packed into the chamber (right).

POST OPERATIVE CARE

After the surgical procedure was accomplished, the Isoflurane was stopped and the animals were observed for spontaneous breathing. The animals were extubated after two minutes of regular spontaneous breathing and were kept under close monitoring for 30 minutes before they were sent to their cages.

Buprenorphine *(Reckitt Benckiser plc, Slough, UK)* 0.04 mg/Kg IM was used every 12 hours to achieve analgesia. This was done regularly for 48 hours and then as needed, according to a periodic evaluation of the animals by the Animal Health Technicians (AHT). All the animals were given a liquid diet for 1 to 2 days post operatively and then fed with regular food as tolerated. All animals were examined and weighed twice a week by the AHT. None of the animals showed any signs of infection or loss of more than 15% of their pre-operative weight.

POST-MORTEM ASSESSMENT AND PREPARATION

Animal sacrifice and samples extract:

All the animals were sacrificed twelve weeks following the grafting procedure. Butorphanol *(Apothecon B.V., the Netherlands)* 0.3 mg/Kg was given for sedation prior to sacrifice and Pentobarbital *(J. M. Loveridge p.l.c., Southamton, UK)* 150 mg/Kg was then infused through an intraauricular intravenous cannula. After cessation of cardiac pulsation was confirmed by the AHT, the animals were transferred to the operating room. Through a submandibular incision, a sharp dissection was performed to expose the lateral aspect of the bodies of the mandible and an en bloc resection of the portion of the body containing the sample was preformed using bone clippers. On clinical observation, the test samples showed more chamber bulk than the empty chambers (Figures 8, 9). The specimens were immediately placed in sterile containers of 70% alcohol and the containers were clearly marked with, the rabbit's name, sample's identification (test or control), and the operation side (right or left body of the mandible). All the specimens were transported to the *JTN Wong Labs (Centre for Bone and Periodontal Research, McGill University, Montréal, QC)* for further processing.

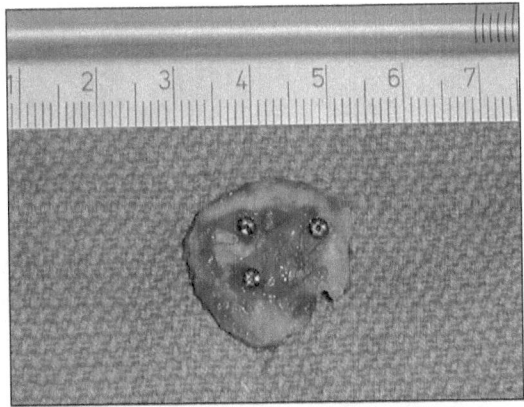

Figure – 8: A postmortem control specimen with screws maintaining the chamber in position and noticeable partial degradation of the membrane.

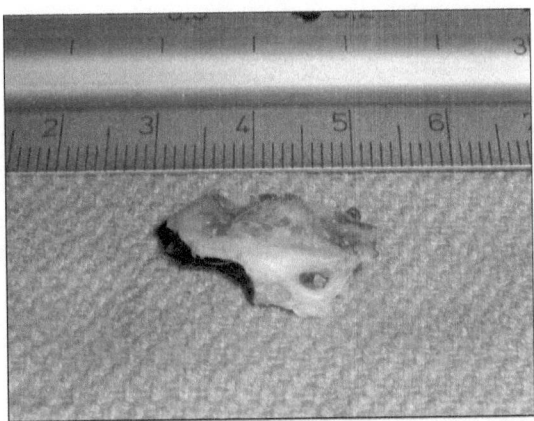

Figure – 9: Lateral view showing the vertical height of a test sample

Micro-CT analysis

All the samples were scanned using a standard desktop micro-CT instrument *(Model 1072, Skyscan, Aartselaar, Belgium)*. The scanner was configured at 100 kV and at 98 µA and images were captured using a 12-bit, cooled CCD camera *(1024 X 1024 pixels)* coupled with a fiber optics taper to the scintillator. The images were then magnified to a 10.94 µm pixel size and the images were sectioned perpendicular to the native bone with a 21.88 µm distance between each cross-section. Each cross-section was reduced to half its size in order to facilitate the analysis, given a voxel size of 21.88 x 21.88 x 21.88 µm3. Next, three-dimensional (3D) rendering models were created for all the specimens, using the 3D Creator and CT-Analyzer software *(SkyScan, Kontich, Belgium)*, and were used for bone volume measurements.

The micro-CT analysis was performed at the Centre for Bone and Periodontal Research in McGill University. The bone volume (BV) is defined as the total bone deposits that were present in the chamber, twelve weeks post chamber's placement. The BV was measured using the 3D Creator software *(SkyScan, Kontich, Belgium)* which created a 3D model from a sequence of two-dimensional images from each sample. On the 3D image the areas of bone were determined and the software *(SkyScan, Kontich, Belgium)* calculated the BV. Bone volume percentage (BV%) is defined as the percentage of bone occupying the total chamber's volume (appendix V). The same technique was used to measure the generated bone height, representing the bone height from the cortical base toward the roof of the chambers (Figure 13).

Histologic preparation and assessment

The specimens were fixated with 70% alcohol and sequentially embedded in Polymethylmethacrylate (PMMA) following the protocol in appendix IV. The histological preparations and the histomorphometric analyses were performed at the *J.T.N Wong Labs (Centre for bone and periodontal research, McGill University, Montréal, QC)*.

Using a microtome the samples were sectioned to produce 4-5 um thick slices. The sections were produced in sagital cross sectional planes through the center of each specimen. These sections were also perpendicular to the outer cortical aspect of the mandible. Two representative sections from the centre of the specimen were chosen and mounted on slides. After deplastification using ethylene glycol, monoethyl ether and acetate respectively for 30 minutes each, staining was applied. The staining was done according to a standardized protocol (see appendix IV). An image of the histological slides that were stained with Von kossa and Toluidine blue was captured using a digital camera connected to a light microscope at 2.5x magnification.

Histomorphometric analysis:

Image-J software (version 1.37v) was used to conduct the histomorphometric analysis. The histological 2 dimensional (2D) slide image was captured and the software was calibrated so that 245.65 pixels equaled 1 mm. The bone deposits were shaded and the particle analyzer feature in the software was used to calculate the bone surface area (BSA). The BSA percentage (BSA%) represents the percentage of bone occupying the total chamber's surface area in 2D.

CHAPTER THREE
EXPIREMENT RESULTS

CLINICAL COURSE

Following the surgeries, all the animals resumed their regular diet on time, and none had any local or systemic complications. Moreover, twelve weeks after the grafting procedures all of the eleven animals were sacrificed as per the experiment protocol. The following section represents the results of the Bone Ceramic (BC) group, the empty (E) chamber group, and the differences between the groups.

Gross description:

Upon dissecting the masseter muscle and periosteum off the mandible, the titanium screws were identified, and aided in locating the chambers. The samples were harvested using bone clippers and were trimmed to produce 2x2 cm specimens (Figures 10, 11). Next, the remaining muscle layer and fibrous tissue were grossly dissected from the sample. This uncovered partial degradation of all the PLA/PGA chambers. The screws were remove easily using screw drivers and the specimens were found to be stable in place.

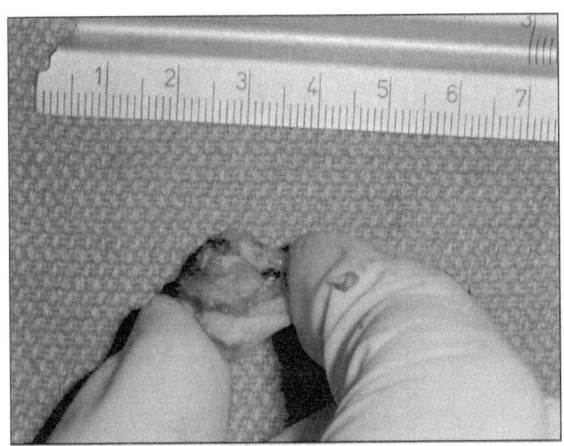

Figure – 10: A post-mortem control specimen showing partial degradation of the membrane

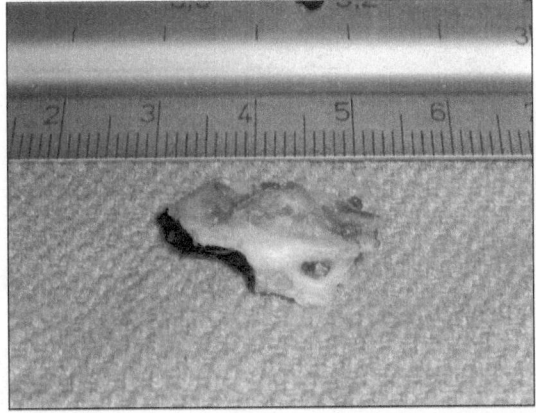

Figure – 11: Lateral view of a test specimen showing the maintained graft volume and vertical height

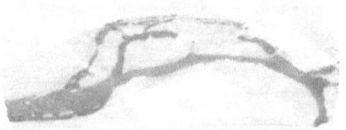

Figure – 12: A grey scale micro CT image of a control sample. The bone (in dark grey hue) is formed in a scattered linear fashion

Micro CT analysis:

The micro CT results of the eleven E samples were the following;

- The (BV%) grew into the chamber ranged from 0.0% to 9.51% with a mean of 3.1% and a standard deviation (SD) of 2.6%.

- The height of bone growth in the chamber (the mean of the original chamber's height was 3.2 mm), ranged from 0.0 mm to 2.0 mm. The mean is 1.1 mm with a SD of 0.6. (Figure 12)

The results of the eleven BC samples were the following;

- The (BV%) grew into the chamber ranged from 11.47% to 37.48%, with a mean of 25.8%, and a SD of 7.3%. (Figure 13).

- The height of bone growth in the chamber ranged from 1.62 mm to 3.15 mm with a mean of 2.6 mm and a SD of 0.4. Table-1 shows the difference between the two groups.

When comparing the BC and the E groups (using paired T test) the following was found:

- BV%: The test group had a BV% mean of 25.8%, and a SD of 7.3% while the control group had a mean BV% of 3.1% and a SD of 2.6%. As a result, the test group demonstrated statistically significant more BV% than the E group, P value < 0.0001.

- The height of bone growth in the chamber: The test group had a mean of 2.6 mm with a SD of 0.4 while the control group had a mean of 1.1 mm with a SD of 0.6. As a result, the test group demonstrated statistically significant more bone height growth in the chamber than the E group, P value < 0.0001. See table-1, graph 1 and 2.

For per specimen values of bone volume, percentage and bone height, see appendix IV

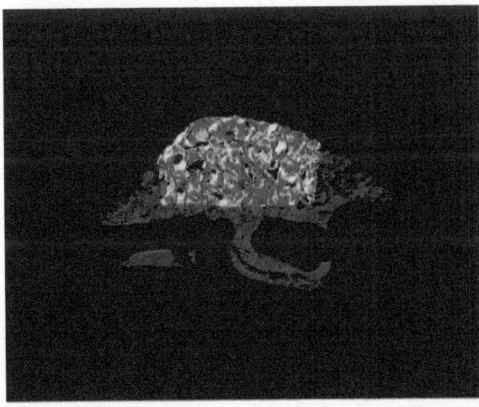

Figure – 13: 3D micro CT image of a test sample. Red (dark) color represents ceramics while white represents bone.

Group	Bone volume % (mean)	Height of Bone (mean)
BC	25.8%	2.6mm
E	3.1%	1.1mm

Table 1: A comparison of the BC and the E group bone volume and height of bone means.

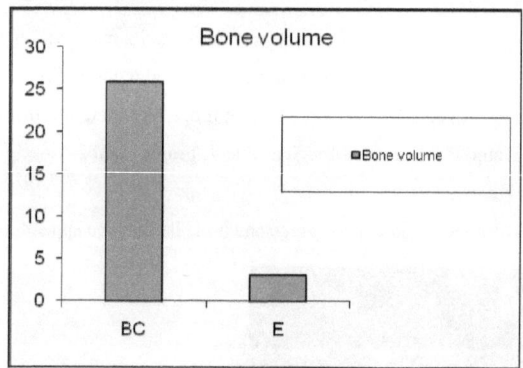

Graph 1: Comparing the mean Bone Volume percentages between the BC (test) and the E (control) groups.

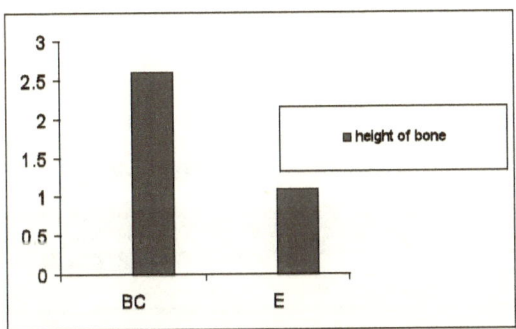

Graph 2: Comparing the mean bone height grown in millimeters between the BC and E groups

Histologic analysis:

Bone trabeculae were identified and noticed to be denser closer to the base of the samples than the roof. The bone tissue looked like immature woven bone with osteoblasts and osteoid deposits. In the BC samples the bone distribution took the shape of multiple semicircles, probably due to the presence of bone at the interparticles spaces (Figure 15). Unlike the BC group, the E samples' bone trabeculae demonstrated multiple linear deposits (Figure 14)

Histomorphometric analysis:

Per sample histomorphometric values can be seen in appendix VI that shows the 11 control (E) samples' examined parameters. These parameters reveal variation in chamber structural maintenance ranging from completely-collapsed chambers to non-collapsed chambers (Figure 14). The BSA% ranged from 0.0% to 15.12% with a mean of 6.23% and a SD of 5.2. Most of the bone distribution occupied the lower third of the chamber.

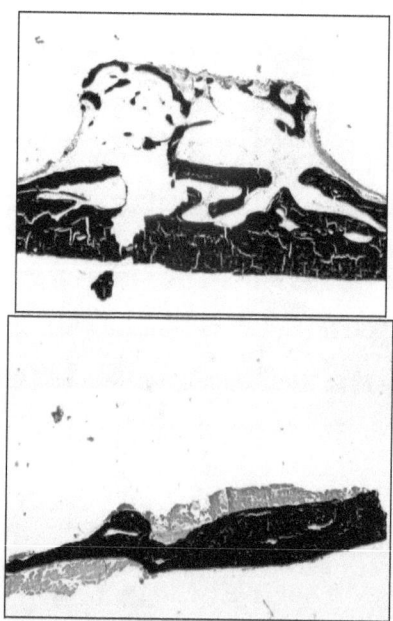

Figure – 14: Two histologic slides of control specimens (2.5 x magnifications) stained with Von Kossa & Toluidine Blue. The figure on top shows a nicely non-collapsed chamber. The bone trabeculae (in black) demonstrated multiple linear deposits. The second image shows another control sample that the chamber got completely collapsed.

In the test group, a total of 11 BC samples were available for histomorphometric examination. The following results were found:
- The BSA% ranged from 7.08% to 33.93%, with a mean of 20.7% and a SD of 7.9. The bone distribution was observed all over the chamber (Figure 15).

Comparing the BC and E groups using paired T test revealed that the BC group had statistically significant higher BSA% than the E group, ($P < 0.0001$) (Graph 3).

Per sample detailed results can be viewed in appendix V.

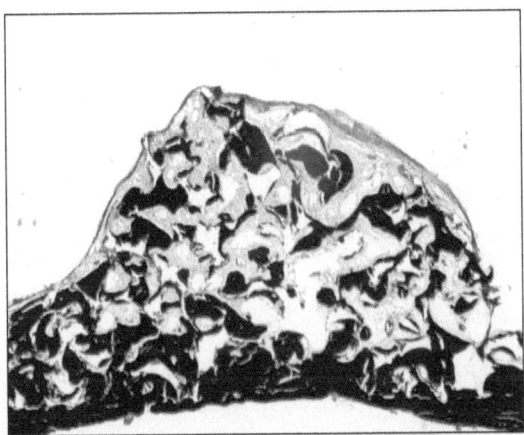

Figure – 15: Histology slide of a BC (test) sample showing bone distribution (black islands) arranged in multiple semicircular deposits. Denser bone aggregates are noticed closer to the base of the chamber than the roof.

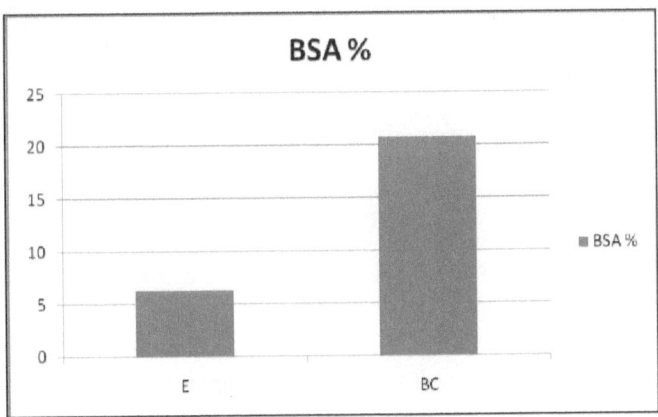

Graph 3: Shows the histomorphometric differnce in BSA% between the test (BC) group and the control (E) group.

Another interesting observation regarding the geometric stability of the collected 22 chambers was identified in the histomorphometric analysis. It was observed that 14 of the 22 chambers (63.6%) maintained their geometric shape (10 were test and 4 were control samples), while 8 of the 22 chambers were collapsed (severe collapse was observed among 7 control samples, and partial collapse was seen in 1 test sample). See appendix V for per sample histomorphometric and chamber geometry analysis.

CHAPTER FOUR
DISCUSSION AND CONCLUSION

THE BIODEGRADABLE MEMBRANE

All the Inion® membranes were covered with fibrous tissue layers that were reflected gently to identify and examine the membranes grossly, and despite being partially degraded, the membranes were identified easily on gross examination.

Inion® membranes are biodegraded by enzymatic hydrolysis that leads to the loss of the membrane's physical properties in 2-4 months after implantation, and complete degradation by 12 months *(Nieminen et al. 2006)*. In our study, it was noticed that after three months of healing, all the membranes had undergone partial degradation.

The main drawbacks of the PLA/PGA membranes are the following:
1. Sensitive handling technique.
2. Time consuming for preparation.
3. Poor chamber geometric stability

THE BONE CERAMIC (TEST) GROUP

Twelve weeks post graft, the BC did not resorb completely and the particles were identified on gross examination. Micro CT and histology showed the homogenous mixture between the BC particles and the bone islands.

The results of this experiment indicated that BC is an osteoconductive material when used as an onlay graft and that PLA/PGA biodegradable membrane was found to be successful in carrying a BC onlay graft.

This study adds more evidence to the literature regarding the osteoconductivity of BC under a PLA/PGA membrane. The bone formed was occupying the interparticle spaces in multiple semicircular deposits (Figure 15).

BC's osteoconductivity has been examined in many studies. As an *onlay*, one study was found that examined BC blocks grafted on sheep's facial skeleton *(Gossain et al 2005)*. Ten sheep were used to compare autogenous cranial (calvarial) bone grafts and HA derived biomaterials (including BC). One year post-implantation, all the blocks were harvested for analysis. The results showed that the cranial bone grafts demonstrated highly significant reductions in volume, while the BC blocks showed higher predictability of graft volume maintenance. In addition, it was found that the bone replacement in BC grafts ranged between 16.4 to 23.9%, which is comparable to the results found in our experiment. Therefore, it was concluded that the graft volume maintenance in onlay BC blocks were highly predictable, whereas that of cranial bone blocks were unpredictable, one year postimplantation.

Aljandan *(2007)* studied cancellous bone onlay graft volumes under PLA/PGA chambers and under titanium chambers. The results showed no significant difference in graft volumes between the PLA/PGA chamber groups and the titanium chamber groups. Aljandan concluded that using either a PLA/PGA chamber or a Titanium chamber is efficient enough to support particulate bone grafts.

Alharkan *(2007)* studied the osteoconductivity of Bio-Oss® onlay grafts under titanium chambers. The mean BV% gained was 18.4%, in which 13.2% of that bone occupied the lower half of the chamber while 5.1% occupied the upper half. In our experiment, the idea of dividing the PLA/PGA chambers to halves was not possible due to the potential geometric changes that could be expected in these biodegradable chambers. However, it was noticed that all the BC samples had bone growth throughout the chamber with a mean BV% of 25.8% and that the bone distribution was denser close to the base of chamber as opposed to the roof area. This might suggest comparable bone distribution when using Bio-Oss or BC as an osteoconductive onlay graft.

Further studies are required to precisely compare the osteoconductivity of Bio-Oss and BC under PLA/PGA chambers.

CONTROL GROUP (EMPTY CHAMBERS)

In our experimental study, the empty PLA/PGA chamber group revealed a BV% mean of 3.1%. Alharkan (2007) placed a Bio-Oss® onlay graft under a titanium chamber on one side of rabbit mandibles, and placed an empty titanium chamber on the contralateral side. He found that the mean BV% under the empty titanium chamber group was 5%. Seemingly, the BV% values found under the titanium chambers in Alharkan's study were higher than those found under the empty PLA/PGA chambers in our study. This is probably due to the superiority of titanium chambers over PLA/PGA chambers in geometric stability; however more precise and controlled studies are required to examine the exact difference.

CONCLUSION

This study confirms that BC is an osteoconductive material when used as an onlay graft under a PLA/PGA biodegradable chamber. This study suggests that this grafting technique could be clinically applied to reconstruct conservative horizontal alveolar bone deficiency. However, further studies are required to assess the quality of this grafting technique to assess the validity for variable defect sizes in different locations in the oral cavity.

Appendix I

Rabbits names, order, surgical sites details.

surgery date	Animal Name	right side	left side	Sacrify date
15-Dec-08	Victory	control	Test	March.30,2009
15-Dec-08	Yale	control	Test	"
15-Dec-08	Kymco	control	Test	"
15-Dec-08	Aprila	control	Test	"
15-Dec-08	Magestic	control	Test	"
17-Dec-08	Cyclone	test	Control	"
17-Dec-08	Boxer	test	Control	"
17-Dec-08	Alléluia	test	Control	"
17-Dec-08	Ducati	test	Control	"
17-Dec-08	Wooler	test	Control	"
18-Dec-08	Taurus	test	Control	"

Appendix II
Design of the titanium chambers and the membrane mold

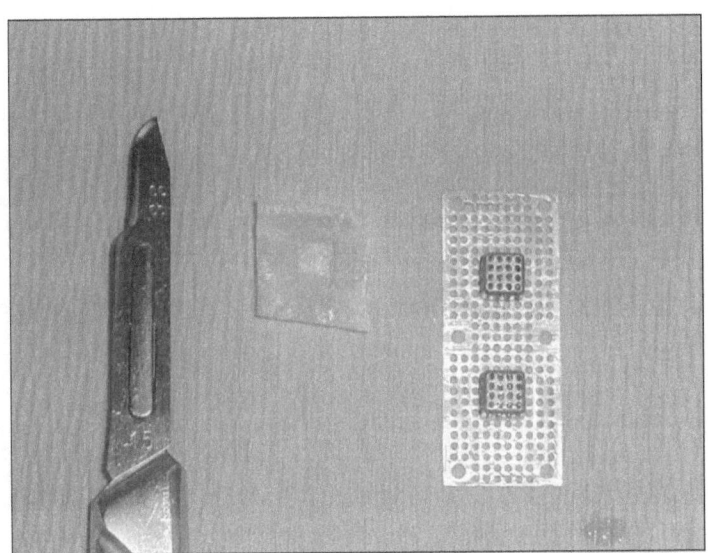

Appendix III
Specimen Preparations and Embedding Protocol

Preparation:

The bone graft specimens were stored sequentially in the following solutions for a minimum of 48 hours:

1- 70 % solution v/v of ethanol (Commercial Alcohols Inc., Brampton, on.) and water for drying.

2- 95 % solution v/v of ethanol and water for drying.

3- 1:1 solution v/v of ether/acetone (JT Baker Inc. Jackson, TN) for degreasing and defatting.

4- Anhydrous ethanol for final drying.

In addition, magnetic stirring at each stage facilitated permeation of each fluid into the bone.

Embedding

Prior to embedding, all specimens were pre-soaked for a minimum of 48 hours in a solution of Polymethylmethacrylate (PMMA) (Aldrich Chemicals, Oakville, On.) inhibited with 10 ppm hyrdoquinone. The PMMA solution was activated with the addition of 3.5g of benzoyl peroxide (Aldrich Chemicals) per liter of PMMA monomer. The specimens in monomer were stored at 4 °C in a refrigerated environment and magnetically stirred.

All specimens were embedded in PMMA. The process of embedding yielded a sample that was encased in a hard, transparent plastic block. In this manner the specimens were well preserved and mechanically stable for a variety of analysis procedures. The liquid monomer was prepared for polymerization as follows:

1) The inhibited (10 ppm methyl hydroquinone) PMMA monomer was activated with the addition of 3.5g of benzoyl peroxide per liter of PMMA monomer.
2) The activated monomer was heated at 55 °C in a hot water bath for approximately six hours. During heating the monomer was stirred each 1/2 hour.
3) When the consistency of the partially polymerized solution was similar to thin syrup and slightly yellow in color, the solution was removed from the hot water bath. Upon removal the solution was cooled under tap water and stored at 1 °C.

Appendix IV
Micro CT Results

Animal Name	Side - sample	Ceramic + Bone (mm3)	Ceramic Only (mm3)	Bone Vol. Only (mm3)	Template (4.5x4.5x3.2mm)	BV/TV (%)	Bone Height (mm)
Victory	right_control	0.66	0	0.66	64.8	1.02%	0.78
Victory	left_test	14.49	1.38	13.11	64.8	20.23%	1.62
Yale	right_control	6.16	0	6.16	64.8	9.51%	2
Yale	left_test	32.65	8.36	24.29	64.8	37.48%	3.15
Kymco	right_control	0.51	0	0.51	64.8	0.79%	0.8
Kymco	left_test	24.85	4.21	20.64	64.8	31.85%	2.88
Aprila	right_control	2.36	0.04	2.32	64.8	3.58%	0.48
Aprila	left_test	26.95	7.89	19.06	64.8	29.41%	2.55
Magestic	right_control	1.28	0	1.28	64.8	1.98%	1.42
Magestic	left_test	23.8	8.1	15.7	64.8	24.23%	2.75
Cyclone	right_test	10.35	2.92	7.43	64.8	11.47%	2.45
Cyclone	left_control	0	0	0	64.8	0.00%	0
Boxer	right_test	24.54	8.2	16.34	64.8	25.22%	2.18
Boxer	left_control	1.9	0.01	1.89	64.8	2.92%	1.65
Alléluia	right_test	23.7	7.67	16.03	64.8	24.74%	2.65
Alléluia	left_control	2.23	0.14	2.09	64.8	3.23%	1.32
Ducati	right_test	20	5.1	14.9	64.8	22.99%	2.99
Ducati	left_control	3.25	0	3.25	64.8	5.02%	1.21
Wooler	right_test	32.31	9.65	22.66	64.8	34.97%	2.95
Wooler	left_control	2.97	0	2.97	64.8	4.58%	1.68
Taurus	right_test	24.84	10.65	14.19	64.8	21.90%	2.58
Taurus	left_control	1.11	0.01	1.1	64.8	1.70%	1.18

Appendix V
Histomorphometric Analysis results

ID	Def	Slide	Bone Surface Area (um2)	standard area (mm2)	% (proportion of bone)	Chamber geometry
Alleluia	TR	ATR	4126685.3	14400000	28.66	Intact chamber
Alleluia	CL	ACL	1684330.71	14400000	11.70	Intact chamber
Aprila	Control-right	ApCR	220819.28	14400000	1.53	Collapsed
Aprila	Test-Left	ApTL	2371889.22	14400000	16.47	Intact chamber
Boxer	TR	BTR	3211386	14400000	22.30	part Collapsed
Boxer	CL	BCL	763527.68	14400000	5.30	Collapsed
cyclone	TR	CTR	1226931.27	14400000	20.58	Intact chamber
cyclone	CL	CCL	2963214.55	14400000	8.52	Collapsed
Ducati	TR	DTR	4281625.71	14400000	29.73	Intact chamber
Ducati	CL	DCL	1582093.39	14400000	10.99	Intact chamber
Kimco	Control-right	KCR	0	14400000	0	collapsed
Kimco	Test-Left	KTL	2000966.21	14400000	13.90	Intact chamber
Magestic	Control-right	MCR	569476.9	14400000	3.95	Collapsed
Magestic	Test-Left	MTL	4886627.16	14400000	33.93	Intact chamber
Taurus	TR	TTR	2978558.49	14400000	20.68	Intact chamber
Taurus	CL	TCL	320721.65	14400000	2.23	all collapsed
Victory	Control-right	VCR	0	14400000	0	all collapsed
Victory	Test-Left	VTL	3081296.16	14400000	21.40	Intact chamber
Wooler	TR	WTR	1953933.7	14400000	13.57	Intact chamber
Wooler	CL	WCL	1320662.71	14400000	9.17	Intact chamber
Yale	Control-right	YCR	2176587.58	14400000	15.12	Intact chamber
Yale	Test-Left	YTL	1019120.98	14400000	7.08	Intact/angled cut

REFERENCES:

Abernathy W, McDaniel M, Edwards R, Kiely K, Frazier D. Nonmetallic fixation in elective maxillofacial surgery. AORN J. 2000;71(1):193-8

Adeyemo WL, Reuther T, Bloch W, Korkmaz Y, Fischer JH, Zöller JE, Kuebler AC. Influence of host periosteum and recipient bed perforation on the healing of onlay mandibular bone graft: an experimental pilot study in the sheep. Oral Maxillofac Surg. 2008;12(1):19-28.

Agarwal S, Gupta A, Grevious M, Reid RR. Use of resorbable implants for mandibular fixation: a systematic review. J Craniofac Surg. 2009;20(2):331-9

Albrektsson, T. and C. Johansson, Osteoinduction, osteoconduction and osseointegration. Eur. Spine J. 2001;10:96-101

Alharkan A. Is Bio-Oss an osteoconductive material when used as an onlay bone substitute? An experimental study in the mandible of the rabbit. Faculty of Dentistry, M.Sc Thesis; McGill University; 2007.

Aljandan B. The efficacy of biodegradable mesh as a fixation device for support of autogenous onlay bone graft: A radiographic and histomorphometric analysis., Faculty of Dentistry,. M.Sc Thesis, McGill University; 2007.

Almasri M., Altalibi M. Efficacy of reconstruction of alveolar bone using an alloplastic hydroxyapatite tricalcium phosphate graft under biodegradable chambers. British J of Oral Max Fac surg. 2011;49:469–473

Alonso, N., Machado de Almeida O, Jorgetti V, Amarante MT. Cranial versus iliac onlay bone grafts in the facial skeleton: a macroscopic and histomorphometric study. The J of Craniomaxillofac Surg. 1995;6(2):113-118.

Bahr W, Stricker A, Gutwald R, Wellens E. Biodegradable osteosynthesis material for stabilization of midface fractures: experimental investigation in sheep. J Craniomaxillofac Surg 1999; 27: 51–57.

Barber HD and Betts. Rehabilitation of maxillofacial trauma patients with dental implants. Implant Dentistry.1993;2:191-3

Bartee BK. A membrane and graft technique for ridge maintenance using high-density polytetrafluoroethylene membrane (n-PTFE) and hydroxylapatite: report of four cases. Tex Dent J. 1995;112(5):7-11

Bartee BK, Carr JA. Evaluation of a high-density polytetrafluoroethylene (n-PTFE) membrane as a barrier material to facilitate guided bone regeneration in the rat mandible. J Oral Implantol. 1995;21(2):88-95

Bartee BK.A simplified technique for ridge preservation after tooth extraction.Dent Today. 1995;14(10):62-7

Bartee BK. The use of high-density polytetrafluoroethylene membrane to treat osseous defects: clinical reports.Implant Dent. 1995;4(1):21-6

Bohner M. Reactivity of calcium phosphate cements. J Mater Chem. 2007;17:3980-6

Bos RRM, Boering G, Rozema FR. Resorbable poly (L-lactide)plates and screws for the fixation of zygomatic fractures. J Oral Maxillofac Surg 45:751, 1987

Bouwman JP, Tuinzig DB. Biodegradable osteosynthesis in mandibular advancement: a pilot study. Br J Oral Maxillofac Surg 1999; 37: 6–10.

Boyne PJ. The evolution of guided tissue regeneration, alveolar bone grafting. Oral Maxillofac. Surg. Clin. North Am 2001;13(3):397.

Burstein FD, Ariyan S, Chicarilli Z, Canalis RF The effect of periosteal preservation on osteogenesis in a canine rib autograft model: tetracycline fluorescence incident photometry. J Craniofac Surg. 1994; 5:161–71

Buser D, Dula K, Belser U, Hirt HP, Berthold H. Localized ridge augmentation using guided bone regeneration. 1. Surgical procedure in the maxilla.Int J Perio Resto Dent. 1993;13(1):29-45

Buser D, Dula K, Belser UC, Hirt HP, Berthold H.Localized ridge augmentation using guided bone regeneration. II. Surgical procedure in the mandible. Int J Perio Resto Dent. 1995;15(1):10-29

Buser D, Dula K, Hirt HP, Schenk RK.Lateral ridge augmentation using autografts and barrier membranes: a clinical study with 40 partially edentulous patients.J Oral Maxillofac Surg. 1996;54(4):420-32

Carlson ER, Marx RE. Part II. Mandibular reconstruction using cancellous cellular bone grafts.J Oral Maxillofac Surg. 1996;54(7):889-97

Chacon GE, Ellis JP, Kalmar JR, McGlumphy EA Using resorbable screws for fixation of cortical onlay bone grafts: an in vivo study in rabbits. J Oral Maxillofac Surg. 2004;62(11):1396-402

Chen NT, Glowacki J, Bucky LP, Hong HZ, Kim WK, Yaremchuk MJ. The roles of revascularization and resorption on endurance of craniofacial onlay bone grafts i the rabbit. Past. Reconstr. Surg. 1994;93(4):714-722.

Cohen SR, Holmes RE, Amis P, Fitchner H, Shusterman EM. Tacks: a new technique for craniofacial fixation. J Craniofac Surg. 2001;12(6):596-602

Constantz BR, Barr BM, Ison IC, Fulmer MT, Baker J, McKinney L, et al. Histological, chemical, and crystallographic analysis of four calcium phosphate cements in different rabbit osseous sites. J Biomed Mater Res. 1998;43(4):451-61

Cox T, Kohn MW, Impelluso T. Computerized analysis of resorbable polymer plates and screws for the rigid fixation of mandibular angle fractures. J Oral Maxillofac Surg. 2003;61(4):481-7

Dahlin C, Linde E. Healing of bone defects by guided tissue regeneration. Plast Reconstr Surg. 1988; 81:672-676

Damien JD and Parsons JR. Bone graft and bone graft substitutes: A review of current technology and applications. J. Appl. Biomater. 1991;2:187

Elhakim M. Autogenous onlay bone grafts to the mandible : an experimental evaluation of graft cellularity and embryonic origin. Faculty of Dentistry. McGill University; 2006

Edwards RC, Kiely KD, Eppley BL. Fixation of bimaxillary osteotomies with resorbable plates and screws: experience in 20 consecutive cases. J Oral Maxillofac Surg. 2001;59(3):271-6

Edwards RC, Kiely KD, Eppley BL. The fate of resorbable poly - L-lactic-polyglycolic acid (LactoSorb) bone fixation devices in orthognathic surgery. J Oral Maxillofac Surg. 2001;59 (1):19-25

Edwards RC, Kiely KD, Eppley BL. Resorbable fixation techniques for genioplasty. J Oral Maxillofac Surg. 2000;58(3):269-72

Edwards RC, Kiely KD. Resorbable fixation of Le Fort(I) osteotomies. J Craniofac Surg 1998;9: 210–214

Ellinger RF, Nery EB, Lynch KL. Histological assessment of periodontal osseous defects following implantation of hydroxyapatite and biphasic calcium phosphate ceramics: a case report. Int J Periodontics Restorative Dent. 1986;6(3):22-33

Eppley BL, Morales L, Wood R, Pensler J, Goldstein J, Havlik RJ, et al. Resorbable PLLA-PGA plates and screw fixation in pediatric craniofacial surgery: clinical experience in 1883 patients. Plast Reconstr Surg. 2004;15;114(4):850-6

Eppley BL. Use of a resorbable fixation technique for maxillary fractures. J Craniofac Surg. 1998;9(4):317-21

Eppley BL, Sadove AM, Havlik RJ. Resorbable plate fixation in pediatric craniofacial surgery. Plast Reconstr Surg. 1997;100(1):1-7

Eppley BL, Prevel CD. Non-metallic fixation in traumatic midfacial fractures. J Craniofac Surg. 1997;8(2):103

Eppley BL, Reilly M. Degradation characteristics of PLLA-PGA bone fixation devices. J Craniofac Surg. 1997;2:116

Enislidis G, Pichorner S, Kainberger F. LactoSorb panel and screws for repair of large orbital floor defects. J Craniomaxillofac Surg 1997;25:316

Fearon JA. Rigid fixation of the calvaria in craniosynostosis without using "rigid" fixation. Plast Reconstr Surg. 2003;111(1):27-38

Ferretti C, Reyneke JP. Mandibular sagittal split osteotomies fixed with biodegradable or titanium screws: a prospective, comparative study of postoperative stability. Oral Surg Oral Med Oral Pathol Oral Radiol Endod. 2002;93(5):534-7

Fleckenstein KB, Cuenin MF, Peacock ME, Billman MA, Swiec GD, Buxton TB, Singh BB, McPherson JC 3rd. Effect of a hydroxyapatite tricalcium phosphate alloplast on osseous repair in the rat calvarium. J Periodontol 2006 Jan;77(1):39-45.

Fonseca, R.J., Nelson JF, Clark PJ, Frost DE, Olson RA. Revascularization and healing of onlay particulate autologous bone grafts in primates. J. Oral Surgery. 1980;38:572.

Froum SJ, Wallace SS, Cho SC, Elian N, Tarnow DP. Histomorphometric comparison of a biphasic bone ceramic to anorganic bovine bone for sinus augmentation: 6- to 8-month postsurgical assessment of vital bone formation. A pilot study. Int J Periodontics Restorative Dent. 2008;28(3):273-81

Fujita R, Yokoyama A, Kawasaki T, Kohgo T. Bone augmentation osteogenesis using hydroxyapatite and beta tricalcium phosphate blocks. J Oral Maxillofac Surg. 2003;61(9):1045-53

Gosain AK, Song L, Riordan P, Amarante MT, Kalantarian B, Nagy PG, et al: Par 1: a one year study of osteoinduction in hydroxyapatite derived biomaterial in an adult sheep model. Plas Reconst Surg. 2002;109:619

Gosain AK, Liansheng S, Paul R, Amarante MT, Nagy PG, Wilson CR, et al: A 1 year study of osteoinduction in hydroxyapatite-derived biomaterials in an adult sheep model: III. Comparison with autogenous bone graft for facial augmentation. Plas Reconst Surg. 2005;116:1044

Gosain AK, Paul A, Liansheng S, Amarante MT, Nagy PG, Wilson CR, et al. A 1 year study of osteoinduction in hydroxyapatite-derived biomaterial in an adult sheep model:

part II. Bioengineering implants to optimize bone replacement in reconstruction of cranial defects. Platic reconstructive surgery. 2004; 114: 1155.

Hans P, Dieter R, Bendex J. Muhling.poly(L lactide): along term degradation study in vivo part (III) Analytical characterization Biomaterials. 1993;14(4):291-8

Hallman M, Sennerby L, Lundgren S. A clinical and histologic evaluation of implant integration in the posterior maxilla after sinus floor augmentation with autogenous bone, bovine hydroxyapatite, or a 20:80 mixture. Int J Oral Maxillofac Implants. 2002;17(5):635-43.

Imbronito AV, Scarano A, Orsini G, Piattelli A, Arana-Chavez VE. Ultrastructure of bone healing in defects grafted with a copolymer polylactic/polyglycolic acids. J Biomed MaterRes A. 2005;74(2):215-21

Imbronito AV, Todescan JH, Carvalho CV, Arana-Chavez VE. Healing of alveolar bone in resorbable and non resorbable memrane-protected defects. A hitology pilot study in dogs. Int J Oral Maxillofac Implants. 2002;17(4):467-72

Inion GTR biodegradable membrane. www.citagenix.com

Jensen SS, Broggini N, Hjørting-Hansen E, Schenk R, Buser D. Bone healing and graft resorption of autograft, anorganic bovine bone and beta-tricalcium phosphate. A histologic and histomorphometric study in the mandibles of minipigs. Clin Oral Implants Res. 2006;17(3):237-43

Jensen S, Aaboe M, Pinholt E, Hjørting-Hansen E, Melsen F, Ruyter E. Tissue reaction and material characteristics of four bone substitutes. The International Journal of Oral and Maxillofacial Implants. 1996; 11: 55-66

Jensen OT, Shulman LB, Block MS, Iacono VJ. Report of the sinus concensus conference of 1996. The int J Oral Maxillofac Imp. 1998;13:11-32

Johansson B, Grepe A, Wannfors K, Hirsch JM. A clinical study of changes in the volume of bone grafts in the atrophic maxilla. Dentomaxillofac Radio 2001 May;30(3):157-61.

Karring, T., Nyman, S., Gottlow, J. & Laurell, L. Guided tissue regeneration – animal and human studies. Periodontology 2000;1:26-35.

Kinoshita Y, Kirigakubo M, Kobayashi M, Tabata T, Shimura K, Ikada Y. Study on the efficacy of biodegradable poly(L-lactide) mesh for supporting transplanted particulate cancellous bone and marrow: experiment involving subcutaneous implantation in dogs. Biomaterials 1993 Aug;14(10):729-36

Kinoshita Y, Kobayashi M, Hidaka T, Ikada Y. Reconstruction of mandibular continuity defects in dogs using poly (L-lactide) mesh and autogenic particulate cancellous bone and marrow: preliminary report. J oral maxillofac surg 1997 Jul;55(7):718-23; discussion 723-4.

Kontio R, Ruuttila P, Lindroos L, Suuronen R, Salo A, Lindqvist C, et al.
Biodegradable polydioxanone and poly(l/d)lactide implants: an experimental study on peri-implant tissue response. Int J Oral Maxillofac Surg 2005;34:766-76.

Kostopoulos L, and Karring, T. Guided bone regeneration in mandibular defects in rats using a bioresorbable polymer. Clinical Oral Implant Research 1994;5: 66-74

Kostopoulos, L. & Karring T. Role of periosteum in the formation of jaw bone. An experiment in the rat. Journal of Clinical Periodontology. 1995;22: 247-254

Landes CA, Kriener S .Resorbable plate osteosynthesis of sagittal split osteotomies with major bone movement. Plast Reconstr Surg. 2003;111(6):1828-40.

Landes CA, Kriener S, Menzer M, Kovacs AF. Resorbable plate osteosynthesis of dislocated or pathological mandibular fractures: a prospective clinical trial of two amorphous L-/DL lactide copolymer 2-mm miniplate systems. Plast Reconstr Surg. 2003;111(2):601-10

Leonetti JA, Koup R. Localized maxillary ridge augmentation with a block allograft for dental implant placement: case reports. Implant Dent 2003;12(3):217-26.

Li S, .McCarthy S. Further investigations on the hydrolytic degradation of poly (DL-lactide), Biomaterials. 1997;20 (1):35-44

Lu M, and Rabie A. Quantitative assessment of early healing of intramembranous and endochondral autogenous bone grafts using micro-computed tomograpgy and Q-win image analyzer. Int. J. Oral Maxillofac. Surg, 2004.;33:369-376.

Matsumoto MA, Filho HN, Padovan LE, Kawakami RY, De Assis Taveira LA. Tissue response to poly-L-lactide acid-polyglycolic acid absorbable screws in autogenous bone grafts: a histologic morphological analysis. Clin Oral Implants Res. 2005;16(1):112-8

McAllister BS, Haghighat K. Bone augmentation techniques. J Periodontol. 2007;78(3):377-96

Meadows CL, Gher ME, Quintero G, Lafferty TA. A comparison of polylactic acid granules and decalcified freeze-dried bone allograft in human periodontal osseous defects. J Periodontol 1993;64:103-9.

Metzger DS, Driskell TD, Paulsrud JR. Tricalcium phosphate ceramic: a resorbable bone implant. Review and current status. J. Am. Dent. Assoc. 1982;105:1035

Mollaoglu N, Cetiner S, Alpaslan C, Gultekin SE, Alpar R. The early tissue response to titanium and LactoSorb screws. Dent Traumatol. 2003;19(3):139-44

Marx RE, Shellenberger T, Wimsatt J, Correa P. Severely resorbed mandible: predictable reconstruction with soft tissue matrix expansion (tent pole) grafts. J Oral Maxillofac Surg. 2002;60(8):878-88

Meningaud JP, Poupon J, Bertrand JC, Chenevier C, Galliot-Guilley M, GuilbertF. Dynamic study about metal release from titanium miniplates in maxillofacial surgery. Int J Oral Maxillofac Surg. 2001;30(3):185-8.

Mainil-Varlet P, Rahn B, Gogolewski S. Long-term in vivo degradation and bone reaction to various polylactides (One-year results). Biomaterials. 1997;18(3):257-66.

Magnusson I, Batich C, Collins BR. New attachment formation following controlled tissue regeneration using biodegradable membranes. J Periodont. 1988;59:1-6

Moghadam H, Sándor G, Holmes H, Clokie C. Histomorphometric Evaluation of Bone Regeneration Using Allogeneic and Alloplastic Bone Substitutes. Journal of Oral and Maxillofacial Surgery. 2004; 62:202-213

Moy PK, Aghaloo TL. Which hard tissue augmentation techniques are the most successful in furnishing bony support for implant placement? Int J Oral Maxillofac Implants. 2007;22 Suppl:49-70

Nakadate M, Amizuka N, Li M, Freitas PH, Oda K, Nomura S, Uoshima K, Maeda T. Histological evaluation on bone regeneration of dental implant placement sites grafted with a self-setting alpha-tricalcium phosphate cement. Microsc Res Tech. 2008;71(2):93-104.

Nieminen T, Rantala I, Hiidenheimo I, Keränen J, Kainulainen H, Wuolijoki E, Kallela I, et al. Degradative and mechanical propertiesof novel resorbable plating system during a 3 year follow up in vivo and in vitro. J Mater Sci Mater Med. 2008;19(3): 1155-63

Norton MR, Odell EW, Thompson ID, Cook RJ. Efficacy of bovine bone mineral for alveolar augmentation; a human histologic study. Clin Oral Implants Res. 2003;14(6): 775-83

Quereshy FA, Goldstein JA, Goldberg JS, Beg Z. The efficacy of bioresorbable fixation in the repair of mandibular fractures: an animal study.J Oral Maxillofac Surg. 2000; 58 (11):1263-9

Ozaki, W. and S.R. Buchman, Volume maintenance of onlay bone grafts in the craniofacial skeleton: micro-architecture versus embryologic origin. Past. Reconstr. Surg., 1998;102(2):291-299

Ozaki W, Buchman SR, Goldstein SA, Fyhrie DP. A comparative analysis of the microarchitecture of cortical membranous and cortical endochondral onlay bone grafts in the craniofacial skeleton. Past. Reconstr. Surg., 1999;104(1):139-147.

Persons BL, Wong GB. Transantral endoscopic orbital floor repairusing resorbable plate. J Craniofac Surg. 2002;13(3):483-8

Pineda LM, Busing M, Meinig RP, Gogolewski S. Bone regeneration with resorbable polymeric membranes. III. Effect of poly (L-lactide) membrane pore size on the bone healing process in large defects. J Biomed Mater Res. 1996;31(3):385-94

Pollick S, Shors EC, Holmes RE, Kraut RA. Bone formation and implant degradation of coralline porous ceramics placed in bone and ectopic sites. J Oral Maxillofac Surg. 1995 Aug;53(8):915-22

Rimondini L, Nicoli-Aldini N, Fini M, Guzzardella G, Tschon M, Giardino R. In vivo experimental study on bone regeneration in critical bone defects using an injectable biodegradable PLA/PGA copolymer. Oral Surg Oral Med Oral Pathol Oral Radiol Endod. 2005;99(2):148-54

Roberts WE, Smith RK, Zilberman Y, Mozsary PG, Smith RS. Osseous adaptation to continuous loading of rigid endosseous implants. Am J Orthod 1984 Aug;86(2):95-111.

Rosenthal, A.H. and S.R. Buchman, Volume maintenance of inlay bone grafts in the craniofacial skeleton. Pastic and reconstructive surgery, 2003;112(3):802-811.

Schenk R. Bone regeneration: Biological basis. In: Buser D, Dahlin C, Schenk RK (eds). Guided Bone Generation in Implant Dentistry. Chicago: Quintessence, 1994;49-100.

Schmid J, Hammerle CHF, Fluckiger L, Winkler JR, Olah AJ, Gogolewski S, Lang NP. Blood-filled spaces with and without filler materials in guided bone regeneration. A comparative experimental study in the rabbit using bioresorbable membranes. Clin Oral Imp Res. 1997;8:75-81

Schmid, J. Wallkamm, B., Hammerle, C.H.F., Gogolewski, S, Lang, N.P. The significance of angiogenesis in guided bone regeneration. A case report of a rabbit experiment. Clin Oral Imp Res. 1997;8:244-248

Schmidt BL, Perrott DH, Mahan D, Kearns G. The removal of plates and screws after LeFort I osteotomy. J Oral Maxillofac Surg 1998;56:184

Serino G, Biancu S, Iezzi G, Piattelli A., Ridge preservation following tooth extraction using a polylactide and polyglycolide sponge as space filler: a clinical and histological study in humans. Clin Oral Implants Res. 2003;14(5):651-8

Shand JM, Heggie AA. Use of a resorbable fixation system in orthognathic surgery.Br J Oral Maxillofac Surg. 2000; 38(4):335-7

Shindo ML, Costantino PD, Friedman CD, Chow LC. Facial skeletal augmentationusing hydroxyapatite cement. Arch. Otolaryngol. Head Neck Surg. 1993;119:185

Slotte C, Lundgren D, Burgos PM. Placement of autogenic bone chips or bovine bone mineral in guided bone augmentation: A rabbit skull study. The International Journal of Oral & Maxillofacial implants. 2003;18:795-806

Stal S, Tjelmeland K, Hicks J, Bhatia N, Eppley B, Hollier L. Compartmentalized bone regeneration of cranial defects with biodegradable barriers: an animal model. J Craniofac Surg. 2001;12(1):41-7

Stavropoulos A, Kostopoulos L, Nyengaard J R, Karring T. Deproteinized bovine bone (Bio-Oss®) and bioactive glass (Biogran®) arrest bone formation when used as an adjunct to guided tissue regeneration (GTR). An experimental study in the rat. J of Clin Perio 2003; 30: 636-643

Stavropoulos A, Kostopoulos L, Mardas N, Nyengaard JR, Karring T. Deproteinized bovine bone used as an adjunct to guided bone augmentation (GBA) An experimental study in the rat. Clinical Implant Dentistry and Related Research. 2001; 3: 156-165

Stendel R, Krischek B, Pietila TA. Biodegradable implants in neurosurgery. Acta Neurochir. 2001;143(3):237-43

Straumann Bone Ceramic. www.straumann.ca

Sumi Y, Miyaishi O, Tohnai I, Ueda M: Alveolar ridge augmentation with titanium mesh and autogenous bone. Oral Surg Oral med Oral Pathol Oral Radiol Endod. 2000;89:268

Surpure SJ, Smith KS, Sullivan SM, Francel PC. The use of a resorbable plating system for treatment of craniosynostosis. J Oral Maxillofac Surg. 2001;59(11):1271-5

Suuronen R. Biodegradable fracture-fixation devices in maxillofacial surgery. I J Oral Maxillofac Surg 1993;22:50–57.

Tharanon W, Sinn DP, Hobar PC, Sklar FH, Salomon J. Surgical outcomes using bioabsorbable plating systems in paediatric craniofacial surgery. J Craniofac Surg 1998;9(5):441–444.

Tuominen T, Jäsmä T, Tuukkanen J, Marttinen A, Lindholm TS, Jalovaara. Bovine bone implant with bovine bone morphogenetic protein in healing a canine ulnar defect. Inter J Ortho, 2001; 25: 5-8

Turvey TA, Bell RB, Tejera TJ, Proffit WR. The use of self-reinforced biodegradable bone plates and screws in orthognathic surgery. J Oral Maxillofac Surg. 2002; 60(1):59-65

Uckan S, Veziroglu F, Soydan SS, Uckan E. Comparison of stability of resorbable and titanium fixation systems by finite element analysis after maxillary advancement surgery. J Craniofac Surg 2009;20(3):775-9

Viljanen J, Kinnunen J, Bondestam S, Majola A, Rokkanen P, Tormala P. Bone changes after experimental osteotomies fixed with absorbable self-reinforced poly-L-lactide screws or metallic screws studied by plain radiographs, quantitative computed tomography and magnetic resonance imaging .Biomaterials. 1995;16(17):1353-8

Von Arx T, Wallkamm B, Hardt N. Localized ridge augmentation using a micro titanium mesh: a report on 27 implants followed from 1 to 3 years after functional loading. Clin Oral Impl Res. 1998;9(2): 123

Wiltfang J, Merten HA, Becker HJ, Luhr HG. The resorbable miniplate system Lactosorb in a growing cranio-osteoplasty animal model. J Craniomaxillofac Surg. 1999;27(4):207-10

Wittenberg JM, Wittenberg RH, Hipp JA. Biomechanical properties of resorbable poly-L-lactide plates and screws: a comparison with traditional systems. J Oral Maxillofac Surg. 1991;49(5):512-6

Yamada, Y., K. Nanba, and K. Ito, Effects of occlusiveness of a titanium cap on bone generation beyond the skeletal envelope in the rabbit calvarium. Clin. Oral Impl. Res. 2003;14:455-463

Yildirim M, Spiekermann H, Biesterfeld S, Edelhoff D. Maxillary sinus augmentation using xenogenic bone substitute material Bio-Oss® in combination with venous blood. A histologic and histomorphometric study in humans. Clinical Oral Implant Res. 2000;11:217-229

Zarb, G. and T. Albrektsson, Osseointegration - a requiem for the periodontal ligament? An editorial. Int. J. Periodont. Rest. Dent., 1991;11:88-91.

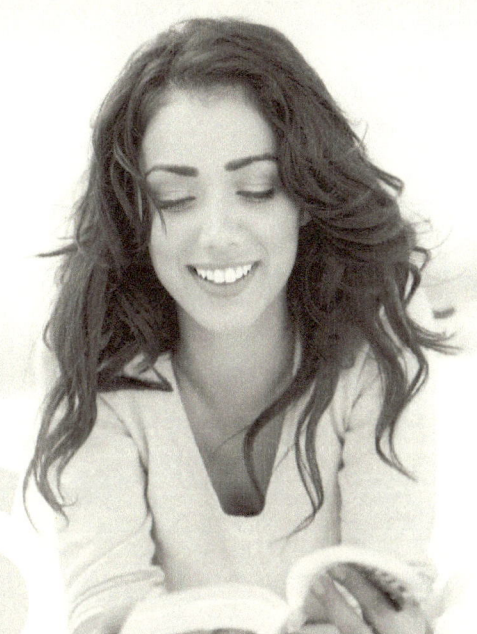

i want morebooks!

Buy your books fast and straightforward online - at one of world's fastest growing online book stores! Environmentally sound due to Print-on-Demand technologies.

Buy your books online at

www.get-morebooks.com

Kaufen Sie Ihre Bücher schnell und unkompliziert online – auf einer der am schnellsten wachsenden Buchhandelsplattformen weltweit! Dank Print-On-Demand umwelt- und ressourcenschonend produziert.

Bücher schneller online kaufen

www.morebooks.de

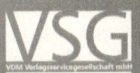 VDM Verlagsservicegesellschaft mbH
Heinrich-Böcking-Str. 6-8   Telefon: +49 681 3720 174   info@vdm-vsg.de
D - 66121 Saarbrücken   Telefax: +49 681 3720 1749 www.vdm-vsg.de

www.ingramcontent.com/pod-product-compliance
Lightning Source LLC
Chambersburg PA
CBHW031543210526
45464CB00003B/1130